SIBO DIET

FOR NOVICES

Enriched Recipes, Foods, Meal Plan & Procedures That Focuses On Boosting Intestinal Health, Weight Management And More

DR. MATEO GABRIEL

Copyright © [Dr. Mateo Gabriel] [2003]. All rights reserved. You can't copy, distribute, or send any part of this book in any way, including by photocopying, recording, or other electronic or mechanical means, without the publisher's written permission first. The only times this is okay are for short quotes in reviews and other legal noncommercial uses.

DISCLAIMER

The information in this book is only meant to be used for general reading. In any way, the author and publisher do not promise or represent that the information in this work is full, correct, reliable, appropriate, or available. This includes any warranties that are expressed or implied. Because of this, you should only rely on this material at your own risk.

This book is not meant to replace professional help. If you have any questions about a subject, you should always get help from a qualified expert. The author and distributor of this book are not responsible for how the information in it is used or abused.

The author's thoughts and feelings are shown in this book. They do not necessarily represent the official policy or stance of any other person, group, employer, or business.

Any third-party material that you can get to through this book is not endorsed or backed by the author or publisher.

The information in this book is correct at the time it was published, after all possible checks. However, the author and distributor are not responsible for any loss, damage, or inconvenience that may be caused by mistakes or omissions.

TABLE OF CONTENTS

CHAPTER ONE 8
   INTRODUCTION TO SIBO DIET 8
      DESCRIBE SIBO 9
      REASONS AND DANGER FACTORS 10
      SIBO SYMPTOMS INCLUDE 11
      IDENTIFYING SIBO 12

CHAPTER TWO 14
   DIET'S FUNCTION IN SIBO MANAGEMENT 14
      WHY EATING COUNTS 14
      THE SIBO DIET'S OBJECTIVES 16
      TYPES OF DIETS FOR SIBO: 17

CHAPTER THREE 20
   DIET LOW IN FODMAPS FOR SIBO 20
      RECOGNIZING FODMAPS 20
      THE LOW-FODMAP DIET'S METHODS 21
      AVOIDABLE FOODS 22
      ITEMS TO CONSUME 23
      PLANS FOR MEALS AND RECIPES 25

CHAPTER FOUR 28
   DIETARY SPECIFIC CARBOHYDRATE (SCD) 28

- PRINCIPLES OF THE SCD 28
- PERMITTED AND PROHIBITED FOODS 29
- SCD IMPLEMENTATION 30
- ACHIEVEMENT STORIES 31
- SCD-COMPATIBLE RECIPES 32

CHAPTER FIVE 34

- DIETARY ELEMENTS 34
  - THE ELEMENTAL DIET: WHAT IS IT? 34
  - HOW SIBO OPERATES 35
  - WHEN TO TAKE INTO ACCOUNT AN ELEMENTAL DIET 36
  - GETTING READY FOR AND FOLLOWING THE 37
  - POSSIBLE DIFFICULTIES AND ADVICE 38

CHAPTER SIX 40

- SIBO'S BI-PHASIC DIET 40
  - OVERVIEW OF THE TWO-PHASIC DIET 40
  - NUTRITIONAL GUIDELINES 41
  - ADDENDUMS 43
  - BRINGING BACK FOODS 44
  - BOOSTING INTESTINAL HEALTH 45

CHAPTER SEVEN 48

- COMBINING SUPPLEMENTS AND PROBIOTICS 48
  - PROBIOTICS' FUNCTION IN SIBO 48
  - SUGGESTIONS FOR PROBIOTICS 50
  - ADDITIONAL ADD-ONS FOR SIBO..........................51
- CHAPTER EIGHT 54
  - ORGANIZING MEALS AND RECIPES 54
    - PLANNING MEALS 54
    - EXAMPLES OF MENUS..56
    - RECIPES SUITABLE FOR SIBOS 58
- CHAPTER NINE 60
  - OVERCOMING PRACTICAL AND SOCIAL OBSTACLES.60
    - OUT TO DINE WITH SIBO 60
    - TAKING DIETARY RESTRICTIONS ON VACATION ...61
    - SHARING YOUR NUTRITIONAL REQUIREMENTS ...63

CHAPTER ONE
INTRODUCTION TO SIBO DIET

A gastrointestinal condition called small intestinal bacterial overgrowth, or SIBO, is brought on by an unusual spike in the number of bacteria living in the small intestine. The process of absorbing nutrients from food that has been consumed occurs in the small intestine, a vital component of the digestive system. On the other hand, when an overabundance of bacteria develops in this area, it may cause several digestive issues and discomfort for those who are impacted.

DESCRIBE SIBO

An imbalance in the small intestine's bacteria population is what defines SIBO. The small intestine typically has a tiny population of bacteria, which are necessary for digestion and the absorption of nutrients. On the other hand, an overabundance of bacteria, especially those that are often found in the colon, can cause the fermentation of undigested carbohydrates, which releases gases like methane and hydrogen. This fermentation process can disrupt the small intestine's regular digestive processes and result in a variety of symptoms.

REASONS AND DANGER FACTORS

SIBO develops as a result of several circumstances. The disturbance of the migrating motor complex (MMC), a sequence of synchronized contractions that comb the small intestine in between meals to remove any remaining germs, is one of the main causes. Intestinal adhesions and specific neurological illnesses are examples of conditions that can damage the MMC and raise the risk of SIBO. Furthermore, anatomical anomalies such as diverticula or strictures in the small intestine can generate areas where bacteria might gather, leading to proliferation.

Compromised immune systems, which can be brought on by illnesses like HIV/AIDS or immunosuppressive drugs, are additional risk factors. Bacteria in the small intestine can also proliferate when there is insufficient production of stomach acid, which can happen while using proton pump inhibitors or when chronic gastritis is present.

SIBO SYMPTOMS INCLUDE

Diagnosing SIBO can be difficult because its symptoms can be varied and overlap with those of other gastrointestinal illnesses. Bloating in the abdomen, excessive gas, diarrhea, and pain in the abdomen are common symptoms. Vitamin and mineral deficits can result from malabsorption of nutrients in people with SIBO. Fatigue, weight loss, and other systemic problems might be signs of these nutritional deficits. Because symptoms can vary widely, medical professionals must do a comprehensive evaluation to differentiate SIBO from other digestive disorders.

IDENTIFYING SIBO

Sufficient identification of SIBO is essential for efficient treatment. The hydrogen-methane breath test is the gold standard for diagnosis. Measuring the amounts of hydrogen and methane gasses in the breath following the consumption of a substrate such as glucose or lactulose is the objective of this non-invasive test. Bacterial fermentation in the small intestine is indicated by elevated amounts of these gasses. Other diagnostic techniques, such as small intestine aspirate or culture, may be used in addition to breath testing, but they are less common and more invasive.

Comprehending SIBO necessitates realizing that it is a complicated gastrointestinal disorder brought on by an overabundance of bacteria in the small intestine.

CHAPTER TWO
DIET'S FUNCTION IN SIBO MANAGEMENT

Dietary decisions have a major impact on the symptoms and course of Small Intestinal Bacterial Overgrowth (SIBO), so controlling the condition with food is essential. A diet that is specifically tailored to the intricacies of SIBO is essential for successful management.

WHY EATING COUNTS

Due to its direct effect on the gut flora, diet is an important factor in the therapy of SIBO. Atypical bacterial overgrowth in the small intestine causes SIBO, which manifests as a variety of digestive problems. The growth of these microorganisms can be stimulated or inhibited by specific food components. Fermentable oligosaccharides, disaccharides, monosaccharides, and polyols, or FODMAPs, for example, might worsen SIBO symptoms by acting as a substrate for bacterial fermentation. However, a well-planned SIBO diet can lessen symptoms and foster an environment that is less favorable to bacterial overgrowth.

THE SIBO DIET'S OBJECTIVES

Reducing the bacterial load in the small intestine, easing symptoms like bloating and abdominal pain, and preventing the recurrence of SIBO are the main objectives of an SIBO-specific diet. Choosing foods that are readily digested, reducing fermentable substrates for bacteria, and promoting general gut health are all necessary to achieve these objectives. Since SIBO can obstruct the absorption of vital nutrients, the diet also attempts to alleviate nutritional malabsorption.

TYPES OF DIETS FOR SIBO:

1. Low-FODMAP Diet: This diet limits the consumption of fermentable carbohydrates, which can lead to bacterial overgrowth in the small intestine due to their poor absorption. The goal of the diet is to lessen SIBO symptoms by cutting less on these substrates. During the early stages of the diet, foods high in fructooligosaccharides (FODMAPS), such as some fruits, vegetables, and grains, are restricted. However, to guarantee adequate nutrition and appropriate food reintroduction, it is imperative to collaborate with a medical practitioner or dietician.

2. The goal of the Specific Carbohydrate Diet (SCD) is to limit complex carbs to lessen the amount of bacteria that ferment in the small intestine. Grain and some sweets, as well as most dairy products, are off-limits in this diet. To starve the microorganisms and encourage gut lining mending, the SCD eliminates these sources of fermentable substrates. It is frequently utilized in conjunction with other holistic methods to treat gastrointestinal disorders, such as SIBO.

3. Elemental Diet: This diet avoids the small intestine entirely by drinking liquid nutrients that have already been partially digested and are hypoallergenic. By offering quickly absorbed nutrients that

leave little behind for fermentation, this method seeks to starve microorganisms. After a brief period on the Elemental Diet to interrupt the SIBO cycle, solid meals are gradually resumed.

4. Diet: The Bi-Phasic Diet emphasizes a step-by-step approach to addressing SIBO by combining components of the Low-FODMAP and SCD. Strict dietary restrictions are usually implemented in the first phase to minimize bacterial overgrowth, and then specific foods are reintroduced in the second phase to determine individual tolerances. A longer-term, more individualized, and sustainable nutrition plan is made possible by this method.

CHAPTER THREE
DIET LOW IN FODMAPS FOR SIBO

RECOGNIZING FODMAPS

Fermentable oligosaccharides, disaccharides, monosaccharides, and polyols are referred to as FODMAPs. These are a class of sugar alcohols and short-chain carbohydrates that the small intestine has trouble absorbing. These substances have the potential to cause the digestive tract to produce more gas and retain more water. Bloating, gas, and abdominal pain are among the symptoms of Small Intestinal Bacterial Overgrowth

(SIBO), which can be made worse by the malabsorption of certain FODMAPs.

THE LOW-FODMAP DIET'S METHODS

One therapy strategy for managing gastrointestinal symptoms linked to disorders such as SIBO is the Low-FODMAP Diet. Reducing the consumption of fermentable carbohydrates and sugar alcohols is the main objective because they may contribute to the expansion of bacteria in the small intestine. The diet's goal is to reduce symptoms and enhance the general digestive health of those who have SIBO by limiting these substances.

The diet is usually used in two stages: the elimination stage, during which foods high in fructooligosaccharides (FODMAPS) are eliminated, and the reintroduction stage, during which particular FODMAPS are progressively added back to determine the individual's tolerance levels.

AVOIDABLE FOODS

Certain foods high in fermentable carbs are advised to be avoided during the elimination phase of the Low-FODMAP Diet for SIBO. These consist of, but are not restricted to:

1. Vegetables high in FODMAPs include broccoli, cauliflower, onions, and garlic.

2. Fruits High in FODMAPs: Watermelon, cherries, mangoes, pears, and apples.

3. Dairy products that include lactose include milk, yogurt, and soft cheeses.

4. High-FODMAP Grains: Products made from wheat, rye, and barley.

5. Pulses and Legumes: Chickpeas, lentils, and beans.

The goal of these limitations is to consume less carbs, which may worsen SIBO symptoms.

ITEMS TO CONSUME

Even if there are fewer high-FODMAP foods available, a low-FODMAP diet for

SIBO can still include a lot of nutrient-dense items. Here are a few instances:

1. Bell peppers, carrots, spinach, and zucchini are examples of low-FODMAP vegetables.

2. Fruits Low in FODMAPs: oranges, kiwis, berries, and grapes.

3. Almond milk, lactose-free yogurt, and lactose-free milk are examples of lactose-free dairy substitutes.

4. Grains Free of gluten: oats, rice, and quinoa.

5. Proteins include tofu, eggs, fish, poultry, and turkey.

These foods can supply important nutrients without aggravating SIBO symptoms.

PLANS FOR MEALS AND RECIPES

Making a meal plan that is both varied and well-balanced is essential for people who are on a low-FODMAP diet. It is critical to investigate and test out various dietary-restrict compliant recipes. A smoothie composed of low-FODMAP fruits, lactose-free yogurt, and a handful of spinach, for instance, might be a breakfast alternative. Steamed carrots and quinoa with grilled chicken would make a satisfying lunch. A little plate of rice and baked fish with roasted zucchini might be dinner. Herbs and spices like ginger, basil, or chives can enhance flavor without ruining your diet.

Careful consideration of food choices is necessary while meal planning for the Low-FODMAP Diet to maintain a well-rounded and fulfilling diet while limiting the chance of causing SIBO symptoms. To develop a customized plan suited to individual requirements and preferences, consulting a certified dietitian with experience in digestive health or a healthcare professional is advised.

CHAPTER FOUR
DIETARY SPECIFIC CARBOHYDRATE (SCD)
PRINCIPLES OF THE SCD

A therapeutic dietary approach called the Specific Carbohydrate Diet (SCD) is intended to manage several gastrointestinal disorders, especially inflammatory bowel illnesses (IBD) such as celiac disease, ulcerative colitis, and Crohn's disease. The SCD was created by Dr. Sidney V. Haas and later made popular by biochemist Elaine Gottschall. It is based on the idea that some carbohydrates negatively affect the gut microbiota and cause inflammation in the intestines.

Eliminating complex carbohydrates—which are believed to provide energy to pathogenic bacteria, yeast, and other microbes in the digestive tract—is the central tenet of SCD.

PERMITTED AND PROHIBITED FOODS

Foods that are permitted and prohibited are crucial in SCD, influencing the dietary options available to people who are trying to recover from digestive issues. The diet emphasizes the ingestion of well-tolerated monosaccharides while excluding disaccharides, polysaccharides, and certain sugars. Lean meats, fresh fruits, non-starchy vegetables, nuts, and some dairy products—like homemade yogurt that has been fermented for at least 24 hours—are among the allowed items. Conversely, foods thought to worsen gut inflammation include grains, legumes, processed sugars, the majority of dairy products, and several fruits and vegetables high in complex carbohydrates.

SCD IMPLEMENTATION

SCD implementation needs to be done carefully because following the dietary recommendations is essential to the program's success. To allow the gut to recover, the first step is to strictly eliminate any foods that don't comply. People can carefully observe the gradual reintroduction of certain meals as their symptoms improve. The process of implementation frequently entails keeping a thorough food log, keeping an eye on symptoms, and seeking advice from medical experts.

People might also need to be aware of any unlisted components and additions in packaged goods that might jeopardize the nutritional integrity of their diet.

ACHIEVEMENT STORIES

Success stories from the SCD community highlight how effective the diet may be in controlling symptoms related to gastrointestinal diseases. Numerous people have reported notable improvements in their overall quality of life, diarrhea, and stomach pain. In addition to providing motivation, these success stories demonstrate the value of tailored strategies because each person's reaction to SCD is unique.

SCD-COMPATIBLE RECIPES

Recipes that are SCD-friendly are essential for sticking to the diet while also providing a varied and pleasurable eating experience. These recipes, which offer alternatives to classic foods that can contain restricted components, frequently concentrate on inventive ways to combine ingredients that are authorized.

Simple dishes like grilled meats and roasted veggies can be made into more complex dinners like baked goodies made with almond flour. The focus lies on discovering the range of foods that comply with the SCD principles, enabling people to develop a dietary regimen that is both enduring and fulfilling.

A dietary intervention that may help with the symptoms of inflammatory bowel illnesses is the Specific Carbohydrate Diet.

CHAPTER FIVE

DIETARY ELEMENTS

THE ELEMENTAL DIET: WHAT IS IT?

A specific nutrition therapy called the Elemental Diet aims to deliver vital nutrients in a form that is easily absorbed. The Elemental Diet calls for the consumption of liquid forms of predigested nutrients, as opposed to whole foods found in standard diets. Those with gastrointestinal disorders, malabsorption concerns, or illnesses like Small Intestinal Bacterial Overgrowth (SIBO) benefit most from this strategy.

HOW SIBO OPERATES

By starving and removing harmful bacteria from the small intestine, the Elemental Diet acts as a therapeutic intervention for people suffering from SIBO. An overabundance of bacteria in the small intestine causes SIBO, which manifests as symptoms like bloating, stomach pain, and changed bowel patterns. By restricting the microorganisms of complex carbohydrates, which serve as their main source of fuel, the Elemental Diet seeks to stop bacterial overgrowth.

WHEN TO TAKE INTO ACCOUNT AN ELEMENTAL DIET

Assessing the degree of digestive problems and the existence of illnesses like SIBO is necessary to decide when to consider the Elemental Diet. The Elemental Diet may be a good alternative for people with SIBO who are resistant to antibiotics or for those who have chronic gastrointestinal problems despite various therapies. It's frequently taken into consideration when traditional therapies don't work or when avoiding prolonged antibiotic use is the main objective.

GETTING READY FOR AND FOLLOWING THE ELEMENTAL DIET

Careful planning and monitoring are necessary when preparing and implementing the Elemental Diet. Individualized plans are usually created by patients in collaboration with healthcare specialists, such as physicians or dietitians, taking into account the severity of their ailment and their nutritional requirements. Consuming a liquid formula comprising simple carbohydrates, vitamins, minerals, and amino acids for a predetermined amount of time—typically two to four weeks—is a common component of the elemental diet. This restricted consumption of elemental nutrients is intended to supply necessary nourishment while reducing the amount of labor that the digestive system must accomplish.

POSSIBLE DIFFICULTIES AND ADVICE

Even though the Elemental Diet has many therapeutic advantages, some people may find it difficult to follow. The diet's liquid format might get boring, and sticking to it for a long time can be emotionally taxing. Aside from that, some people could struggle with social elements of missing regular meals or developing taste aversions. Healthcare professionals frequently provide patients with support and direction to help them overcome these obstacles and find ways to make the process more bearable.

The Elemental Diet is a specific dietary strategy that is essential for treating illnesses like SIBO. It acts as a liquid source of predigested nutrients, which helps reduce the symptoms of small intestinal bacterial development. Integrating the Elemental Diet into a therapeutic regimen for gastrointestinal health requires understanding when to consider it, planning for its implementation, and providing relevant suggestions to overcome any problems.

CHAPTER SIX

SIBO'S BI-PHASIC DIET

OVERVIEW OF THE TWO-PHASIC DIET

A nutritional strategy called the Bi-Phasic Diet was created to treat Small Intestinal Bacterial Overgrowth (SIBO), a disorder marked by an unnatural rise in the number of bacteria in the small intestine. This diet is divided into two phases, each with its own set of nutritional requirements and objectives. The Bi-Phasic Diet's main goals are to starve and lessen the overgrowth of bacteria in the small intestine in the first phase, and then gradually reintroduce specific foods in the second phase to support a healthy gut environment. The goal of this deliberate two-phase treatment is to improve gut health and reduce SIBO symptoms.

NUTRITIONAL GUIDELINES

As the main source of energy for the enlarged bacteria, fermentable carbohydrates are limited in the early phase of the Bi-Phasic Diet, which focuses on a low-fermentation diet. Because they can promote bacterial overgrowth and worsen SIBO symptoms, several forms of carbohydrates, such as FODMAPs (fermentable oligosaccharides, disaccharides, monosaccharides, and polyols), are frequently excluded during this phase of treatment. The intention is to reduce the population of bacteria by establishing an environment that deprives them of their preferred fuel.

The Bi-Phasic Diet's second phase is gradually reintroducing particular foods to vary the diet and promote a balanced, healthful gut microbiome. This stage is critical for maintaining long-term gut health and preventing the recurrence of SIBO. Foods are gradually added back in, enabling people to track their body's reactions and pinpoint potential triggers. The focus switches to a more diversified and sustainable diet that promotes general health and lowers the chance of bacterial overgrowth.

ADDENDUMS

To complement the Bi-Phasic Diet and alleviate any nutritional deficits that may result from dietary restrictions, supplements are essential. During the first stage, supplements could contain minerals that maintain the integrity of the gut lining, antimicrobial drugs to target and reduce bacterial overgrowth, and digestive enzymes to help with food breakdown. To aid in the restoration of a balanced and healthy gut flora during the second phase, probiotics—beneficial bacteria—may be administered. Depending on the severity of SIBO and the unique requirements of each individual, the choice and amount of supplements are frequently customized.

BRINGING BACK FOODS

Following the first restricted phase of the diet, some food groups are gradually reintroduced into the diet during the reintroduction phase of the biphasic diet. This step necessitates closely observing symptoms and responses to pinpoint any meals that can aggravate SIBO or cause discomfort. Foods are gradually reintroduced so people may determine their tolerance and make educated decisions about their diet going forward. This stage involves developing a long-term, sustainable, well-balanced diet that supports digestive health in addition to increasing the variety of foods available.

BOOSTING INTESTINAL HEALTH

The Bi-Phasic Diet places a strong emphasis on promoting general gut health in addition to its food components. Lifestyle choices like stress reduction, regular exercise, and getting enough sleep are crucial for preserving a healthy gut environment. In addition to food, stress-reduction strategies such as mindfulness and relaxation training are frequently suggested. For long-term success in controlling and preventing the recurrence of the illness, it is also essential to address underlying causes that may contribute to

SIBO, such as decreased motility or anatomical abnormalities in the gastrointestinal system. When combined with extensive lifestyle changes, the Bi-Phasic Diet offers a comprehensive strategy for promoting gut health and successfully managing SIBO.

CHAPTER SEVEN

COMBINING SUPPLEMENTS AND PROBIOTICS

PROBIOTICS' FUNCTION IN SIBO

The disorder known as Small Intestinal Bacterial Overgrowth (SIBO) is typified by an unusual rise in the amount of bacteria present in the small intestine. Probiotics help maintain a balanced and healthy gut microbiota, which is essential for controlling SIBO. Probiotics assist in reestablishing the balance in the gut flora, which is a hallmark of SIBO and can cause a variety of digestive problems. Probiotics are live bacteria that give the host health advantages when given in sufficient doses.

When it comes to SIBO, they help control the excess bacterial development in the small intestine and relieve symptoms related to the digestive system as a whole.

According to clinical research, some probiotic strains may be especially helpful in treating SIBO. Bacterial overgrowth can be inhibited and gut flora modulated by strains such as Saccharomyces boulardii, Bifidobacterium breve, and Lactobacillus casei. By posing a competition with pathogenic bacteria for nutrients and adhesion sites in the small intestine, these probiotics prevent the growth of these bacteria. Probiotics can also strengthen the intestinal barrier and stop germs from moving from the small intestine to other areas of the digestive system.

SUGGESTIONS FOR PROBIOTICS

Selecting probiotic strains that have shown effectiveness in clinical trials is crucial when including them in an SIBO management plan. Because Lactobacillus and Bifidobacterium species can help restore equilibrium to the gut microbiota, they are frequently suggested for SIBO therapy. Combinations of these strains—Lactobacillus acidophilus, Lactobacillus casei, Bifidobacterium longum, and Bifidobacterium breve, for example—found in probiotic supplements are frequently seen as advantageous.

It's crucial to remember that different people react differently to probiotics, so experimenting to discover the ideal mix and dosage may be necessary. Speaking with a medical expert, particularly one who has treated SIBO cases, can assist in customizing a probiotic program to a patient's unique requirements and symptoms.

ADDITIONAL ADD-ONS FOR SIBO MANAGEMENT

Certain nutrients can help control SIBO in addition to probiotics by addressing underlying problems and promoting general gut health. One such class of supplements that can help with food breakdown and improve nutrient absorption is digestive enzymes. This is especially important for those with SIBO, as bacterial interference with normal digestive processes can lead to malabsorption, which is a problem.

In certain instances, herbal antimicrobials and antibiotics could also be recommended to lessen the overgrowth of bacteria in the small intestine. When taken with medical advice, these supplements can be a component of a complete strategy for controlling SIBO.

To manage SIBO, supplement integration must be done carefully and under individualized advice. Depending on the individual's unique situation, supplements may or may not be beneficial. To guarantee a safe and customized approach to supplementation, professional supervision is necessary. Probiotics and other supplements can help control SIBO effectively and restore a healthy gut environment when included in a comprehensive treatment strategy.

CHAPTER EIGHT

ORGANIZING MEALS AND RECIPES

PLANNING MEALS

A healthy, well-balanced diet is largely dependent on effective meal planning. It entails giving careful regard to dietary requirements, individual preferences, and lifestyle restrictions. Having a firm grasp of your nutritional objectives is one of the cornerstones of effective meal planning. Whether your objective is to grow muscle, lose weight, or follow a certain diet, it will direct your meal-planning process.

To guarantee that you get a wide range of nutrients, think about including foods from different dietary categories. Lean proteins, entire grains, fruits, vegetables, and healthy fats should all be consumed in moderation. Meal planning is another useful advice. Ideally, you should plan your meals for the entire week. Not only does this save you time, but it also empowers you to make better selections instead of giving in to the allure of quick, less healthful solutions.

Take into consideration portion sizes to avoid overindulging and to keep your calorie consumption under control. It's helpful to become familiar with serving sizes and, if necessary, utilize instruments like food scales or measuring cups. In addition, when it comes to meal planning, flexibility is key. To keep things interesting and accommodate shifting tastes, make allowances for substitutes and adjustments in your meals.

EXAMPLES OF MENUS

Making an example meal plan will make it easier to follow through on your nutritional objectives. A well-designed meal plan considers your taste preferences, nutritional needs, and daily energy requirements. A healthy day could begin, for instance, with a filling breakfast of Greek yogurt, whole-grain oats, and an assortment of fresh fruits.

A slice of fruit or a handful of nuts could make up a mid-morning snack.

A lean protein source, like grilled chicken or tofu, along with a heaping helping of veggies and a complex carbohydrate, like sweet potatoes or quinoa, maybe the main course of lunch. Snacks for the afternoon can be anything as simple as a small dish of cottage cheese or veggie sticks with hummus. Dinner could consist of a modest amount of nutritious grains and a colorful assortment of vegetables together with a meal of fish, lean meat, or plant-based protein.

Always remember to drink enough water to stay hydrated throughout the day. Sustainability and adherence can be ensured by tailoring these meal plans according to nutritional needs, lifestyle circumstances, and individual tastes.

RECIPES SUITABLE FOR SIBOS

Meal preparation presents unique obstacles for individuals suffering from Small Intestinal Bacterial Overgrowth (SIBO). It's important to concentrate on recipes that are kind to the digestive system and support gut health for people who are treating SIBO. Selecting foods that are simple to digest and reducing specific kinds of carbs can be helpful.

Low-FODMAP (fermentable oligo-, di-, mono-saccharides, and polyols) substances can help reduce SIBO symptoms, therefore take into consideration recipes that include them. A tasty breakfast alternative is a low-FODMAP fruit smoothie, including kiwi or berries, blended with lactose-free yogurt or almond milk. This smoothie is SIBO-friendly.

Lean meats, such as chicken or fish, can be the main ingredient in lunch and supper recipes when combined with non-starchy vegetables, such as spinach, carrots, and zucchini. Instead of using high-FODMAP seasonings, you can improve the flavor without aggravating symptoms by using herbs and spices. For people with SIBO, rice or quinoa can be good sources of carbohydrates.

CHAPTER NINE
OVERCOMING PRACTICAL AND SOCIAL OBSTACLES
OUT TO DINE WITH SIBO

Managing social and practical obstacles can be particularly difficult when dealing with particular nutritional needs in a variety of contexts. Eating out while suffering from Small Intestinal Bacterial Overgrowth (SIBO), a disorder characterized by an overabundance of bacteria in the small intestine, is one such situation. People who have SIBO frequently struggle to select healthy meals when they eat out. The difficulty is in coming up with solutions that fit their dietary constraints, such as avoiding specific carbohydrates that can make their symptoms worse. Choosing meals from a restaurant menu requires careful thought, with a focus on finding options that satisfy SIBO-specific dietary requirements while also being palatable.

TAKING DIETARY RESTRICTIONS ON VACATION

Even while traveling is exhilarating, people who follow dietary restrictions may face additional difficulties. Whether it's because of dietary preferences or medical conditions, traveling while following a specific diet necessitates careful preparation. When you have dietary limitations, you must plan for the food selections at your location, bring appropriate snacks, and properly communicate your dietary requirements. Finding accommodating eateries at the destination and navigating the food options at the airport involves careful balancing between exploration and following one's dietary restrictions. A proactive approach is necessary to effectively manage dietary limitations when traveling so that the excitement of discovery is not overshadowed by worries about food compatibility.

SHARING YOUR NUTRITIONAL REQUIREMENTS

Navigating social and practical problems associated with unique eating requirements requires effective communication of dietary demands. To make sure that one's demands are recognized and honored, whether one is managing SIBO or any other dietary limitation, good communication is essential. It's critical to let restaurant personnel or event hosts know about any dietary limitations you may have when dining out or attending social gatherings. This includes stating any dietary restrictions, inquiring about ingredient specifics, and, if required, requesting recipe adjustments. In addition to helping with the practical side of managing dietary demands, fostering open and honest communication among peers also promotes understanding among peers and a supportive social environment.

Managing social and practical obstacles while adhering to particular nutritional needs necessitates a multifaceted strategy. People need to use a mix of preparation, open communication, and research when dealing with the nuances of traveling with dietary restrictions, eating out with SIBO, or effectively communicating their demands.

www.ingramcontent.com/pod-product-compliance
Lightning Source LLC
LaVergne TN
LVHW012324010225
802758LV00010B/633